Reiki II

A Guidebook (2nd Edition)
Now Includes "Reiki With A Twist"™

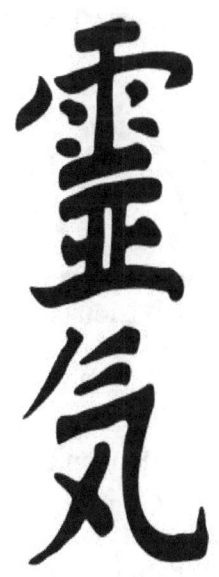

Rev. Kenneth J. Nelan, RM/T, OPoc
Janet C. Soldon, MA, R-LSW, RM/T

Reiki II: A Manual

ISBN: 978-1508975076

Published in the United States by:

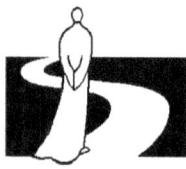

Sacred Wandering / Sacred Path Practitioners
Publishing Division
Glendale, WI.

Printed by: CreateSpace, An Amazon.com Company

For More Information Contact:
Sacred Wandering / Sacred Path Practitioners
c/o Kenneth J. Nelan
5737 N. Sunny Point Rd
Glendale, WI. 53209

http://sacredwandering.com/publishing/

First Printing: 2010

Acknowledgments

All images in this manual are taken from "free source" distributions. There is a general understanding with all Reiki Masters that we all use the same pictures and drawings of symbols that may have originated from Mrs. Takata's school in Hawaii. To the author's general knowledge, there are no copyrights on any of the images in this book and they may be distributed freely. Additionally, many images in this book are originals created by Kenneth J. Nelan. They too may be distributed freely in the interest of common good.

Special Thanks

We would like to thank our many students, who through the years have helped shape our classes with their questions and suggestions. Without any of you we might never have needed such a comprehensive manual. Keep asking your questions; never settle for anything and challenge yourselves daily.

Within This Manual...

About This Manual

This manual has two distinct methods woven together like a fine tapestry. The two methods have been separated using the following headings: The Usui Method, and The Twist™. Any section which does not have a heading does not differ from current Reiki teaching, or is considered common knowledge within the Reiki community.

The Usui Method

The Usui Method sections will be labeled, but will also take up most of this book. The Usui method used today is primarily taken from the teachings brought over from Japan and then modified by Mrs. Takata. It is the information specific to the Usui Shiki Ryoho lineage of Reiki which includes the teachings of Mikao Usui, Chujiro Hayashi, and Hawayo Takata.

Most Reiki practitioners should agree this section is primary to understanding Reiki, its history, and methodologies.

The Twist™

The Twist™ sections will be clearly labeled and shall include information specifically derived from the original teachings of Dr. Usui, and which have, for one reason or another, been lost to the traditional teachings as passed on by Mrs. Takata. These methods have reemerged due in part to efforts of Reiki Masters and Teachers such as Mr. William Rand and Mr. James Deacon. Both have conducted extensive research and study going back to the original teachings of Dr. Usui, much of which has been lost and is slowly being reintegrated into Reiki teachings.

The "Twist" sections may also contain information which is not in keeping with traditional teachings, but has been tested and used in private practice, and through extensive study by the authors has proven to be of great value. It is information congruent with Energywork in general and incorporates real practical information valuable to Reiki practitioners and students.

Reiki With A Twist™ is a Trademark teaching style which was first coined by Kenneth J. Nelan and Janet C. Soldon in their private practice in 2002. It refers to replacing current understanding and information with real practical experience or nontraditional teaching.

Caveat

The information contained in this book is not of a western medical nature, but instead deals with a complementary energy healing technique. Reiki is not a substitute for regular medical care, nor is it to be used as a substitute for emergency services.

At no time should it be implied that the authors are giving medical advice. As always, in case of serious illness, injury, or other condition, consult your own medical practitioner.

By using this book you agree that neither Janet C. Soldon, Sacred Wandering / Sacred Path Practitioners, Kenneth J. Nelan or any affiliates or associates shall in any way be held liable for any misuse of the information contained herein. You are also agreeing to take personal responsibility for your own health and actions as related to the information within this book.

There is no guarantee that by reading this manual you will be accepted by any Reiki program, practitioner, or instructor, or that you will be attuned to the second level of Reiki.

Please seek a qualified and experienced Reiki teacher for your training.

Reiki II

Foreword

The Usui Method

The Five Reiki Principles
Just for today, do not worry.
Just for today, do not anger.
Honor your parents, teachers, and elders.
Earn your living honestly.
Show gratitude to everything.
                    ~ Dr. Mikao Usui

Hopefully by now we have all heard the principles and perhaps we have even learned to incorporate them into our lives, but what do they really mean and why is there such an emphasis and focus on those five lines of prose? We would like to offer you another look at the Reiki Principles.

While reading, keep this in mind: How do you understand the Five Reiki Principles?

Do Not Worry

Many of us have been taught since childhood to anticipate what the day, week, or lifetime holds for us. It is a program running continuously through our subconscious directing us towards a perceived or hoped for outcome. However, what usually happens is that we spend large amounts of time focusing on things that may never happen. It has become a part of our learned nature to focus on those things which will produce positive results for our needs. We begin to expect an outcome for each and every one of our actions and invariably the expected outcome is attached to how we feel about ourselves, those around us, our loved ones, or even our co-workers.

As Reiki practitioners we need to learn NOT to expect an outcome or result of our actions. We are simply tools to draw upon, move, and further enhance the natural energies around us. It is also simply not right to impose our own will over the energy, much less over the intention of our client. When we expect an outcome or result, we often work towards that particular outcome rather than allowing the energy to do what it does naturally, to go where it is needed

Therefore, today we should not worry about anything. If we do not focus on an outcome, then we focus only on our client and their needs or intentions.

What is meant to happen will happen regardless of our desires or actions. We give up control and become that which we move: energy.

Do Not Anger

Are we humans prone to emotional releases? Yes we are. We are human beings and as such are prone to all sorts of emotional responses, not the least of which is anger. Anger can be brought about through repeated frustrations, feeling slighted, disrespected, or wronged. It can also be the direct result of fear.

It is our nature to superimpose other emotions over those which make us feel uncomfortable. Fear, surprise, sadness, and other such emotions which expose our weaknesses, cause us great discomfort and can even be interpreted to threaten our standings with our peers. Society even uses the term "emotional" as a negatively charged word by inappropriately labeling people as "emo". Though originally intended to classify a type of music, the word has become synonymous with those who show their emotions or "wear their heart on their sleeves."

Anger is one of those emotions that is used to cover up, or hide other emotions. It is less threatening to ourselves, and turns the perceived threat outwards as if trying to prove we are not vulnerable. When we display anger, we are really showing that we are unable to deal with the real emotions behind the visceral display of aggression.

As a Reiki practitioner, we must understand and deal with any of our own personal emotions so we do not project those emotions on to our clients or worse; damage or harm someone. We must know who we are inside and deal with those things keeping us from the full knowledge of the self.

And let's face facts: does anyone want to be around someone who is angry or displays aggression? Not really. Those people are usually avoided like the plague, or associated with anger management issues and / or dominance issues.

If I hold myself in check, just for today, and if I become angry, I must deal with it, discover why I feel the need to cover up my true emotions with this anger thing, and move on past the anger towards love for all things and people. The ultimate goal is to view everything around us the same as the energy does; as one and the same thing without boundaries, and without judgment.

Work Honestly

The principle of Working Honestly tells us to keep ourselves in check and to make sure what we are doing does not harm anyone or anything. By working honestly we are ensuring our own well-being as well, as that of our clients.

Remember, above all else, do unto others as you would have them do unto you. Having a good sense of ethics is important.

The principle of Working Honestly tells us to keep ourselves in check and to make sure what we are doing does not harm anyone or anything. By working honestly we are ensuring our own well being as well as that of our clients.

Remember, our clients aren't just those seeking aid, but they are also our students, our families, our friends, and everyone or everything around us.

When we work honestly, we are promoting a different sort of well-being. We are creating an environment of holistic health where everything is bound by the ethical consideration of "Do No Harm".

We are healers. There is no delineation as to who or what we heal, we simply heal.

Respect and Be Kind to All Things

This one should be a given. It is a phrase which has gone through many different interpretations over the vast existence of humanity, but it all boils down to this: "do unto others what you would have them do unto you.[1]"

This is one of those principles which walk hand in hand with the principle of not being angry. Why in the

---

1   New American Bible/ Saint Joseph Edition/No.611/04. Luke 6:31. Boston: Catholic Book Company, 1987. Print.

world would anyone want to treat someone poorly? It is simply unfathomable to think that someone in this world would be so filled with animosity as to be deliberately disrespectful and unkind to others. It is simply beyond comprehension that someone would be anything but kind and gentle.

Respect and be kind to all things is fairly self-explanatory.

I Will Give Thanks For My Blessings

Do we see only those areas we need to improve, or do we also recognize those things we do well? Do we only see that we may not have pleased a client today, or do we see the 5 other clients who were thrilled beyond belief for the services they received? Do you see the glass half full, or half empty? Do you have a positive outlook, or do you focus on those experiences that have kept you down?

I have a special place in my heart for the old saying, "'Tis better to light a candle than curse the darkness[2]", and have discovered in the course of many meditations that this one phrase has profound meaning both literally and figuratively. If there is something which can be remedied, then do so rather than focusing on the fact it existed in the first place.

---

2   A version of this saying was used by John Kennedy, in his acceptance speech to the Democratic Convention, in Los Angeles in 1960: "We are not here to curse the darkness; we are here to light a candle." Who originally coined the phrase is unknown.
<http://www.phrases.org.uk/meanings/207500.html>. 2009. Online.

Even deeper still is the thanks we can give for the darkness. If there existed no darkness would we really understand the light? Would we even have need of a such a thing known as a candle? The darkness then is a balance to the light. Without one, we can never know the other.

By giving thanks for what we have, we recognize there have been moments in our lives when we did not have or had less of what we do now. We learn to appreciate those things, aspects, people or what have you, into our lives. We learn to NOT take things for granted; that they will always be there when we need them. Instead we work towards the positives and improve that which can be improved.

Even those things in our lives which are less than positive can be things for which to be thankful. Everything we do, or every reaction to something we have done teaches us a valuable lesson. If you burn your hand on the stove, it does not become a negative experience unless you continue to dwell on the experience so that it becomes a part of your living fears. Instead it should become a learning moment where we recognize we have learned not to touch a burning stove. Be thankful you have learned the lesson and were then able to move on.

Being thankful does not mean replacing the negative experiences in our lives with a positive outlook, but it instead helps us recognize there really is no positive or negative experience. There exist only the pureness of the experiences. They are neither good, nor bad, but exist to help us grow in this life and move forward on our path. It is our own perceptions of the events which determine how we treat what we view through our own understanding of the world around us.

Be Thankful that you live and are able to feel; that you are able to experience and learn from those experiences. Be thankful you are, and because you are, you will always be.

The simplicity of the Five Principles is perhaps the greatest achievement a Reiki practitioner can ever hope to achieve. They are things to which we should aspire, and help guide our ethical beings on the path to health, wellness, and personal wholeness.

As you travel your path, and read this manual, engage your mind on the possibilities which exist within you. See past the minutia of worry and self-doubt, and experience the fullness of your complete being.

Be Reiki.

About This Book

*A personal note from the authors

Throughout our years of practice and education we have noticed a serious lack of comprehensive teaching on the most basic of Reiki levels – the introductory and Reiki I levels. We have therefore opted to include several review chapters in this book to help refresh and guide those seeking to work on the mental/emotional level of Reiki. Much of what is contained in those chapters may seem redundant, but we have found them necessary to complete the new practitioner's experience.

Reiki II

Chapter 1: Reiki Review

It is somewhat important to understand that Reiki is not owned by any one group or individual. It is not something that can be attributed to any one particular school of thought, or lineage as it is something which is constantly evolving and growing as we grow and evolve within our own existence.

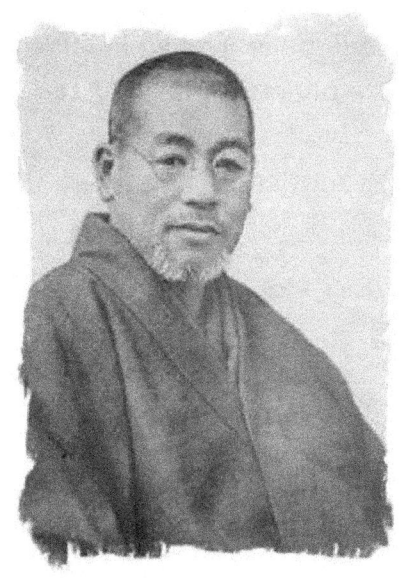

Reiki existed well before Dr. Usui "re"-discovered it's existence, however he is considered by all to be the father of this energy healing modality. Remember, he did not create Reiki, but rather he found ancient scrolls in a Tibetan monastery written in Sanskrit which contained all the mysteries of a healing technique which focused on healing the very core of an individual: their energy.

As the story goes, it was only after he found and translated the scrolls that he did ascend Mt. Kurama to meditate on, and try to understand what he discovered. He did not create the tradition, but merely interpreted the healing modality from ancient wisdom handed down from person to person.

After his twenty-one day fast on the mountain, he came down and began using what he discovered. He didn't start a school, he started to heal others. The Usui school was actually started by his dear friend Dr. Hayashi and not, as some have contended, by Dr. Usui[3].

Dr. Usui taught many people how to heal using this new methodology, but it was Dr. Hayashi who formulated the way in which Reiki is taught today.

The very first thing Reiki teaches us is that all life is connected through a universal flow of energy, or life force, and that this life force can become blocked or flow in excess within an individual, which may cause "dis-ease[4]".

The different bodies are broken down in this way:

---

3   Stein, Diane. *Essential Reiki Teaching Manual An Instructional Guide for Reiki Healers.* New York: Crossing, 2007. Print.

4 The term "dis-ease" is used as a substitute for the word *disease* by individuals and healers in the health and wellness communities. In doing so, they place emphasis on the natural state of "ease" being imbalanced or disrupted, without giving too much focus to a particular ailment.

The Usui Method

The Reiki Precepts

1. The Person Must Ask

Only those who want to be healed can be healed. No one can be healed against their will, or who doesn't want to be healed. It is for that reason the first precept of Reiki is that a person must ask for healing. In asking to for help we open ourselves to the possibility of improved change, growth, and health. When we vocalize and hear ourselves say, "I want to change where I am; I want to change how I am doing something," we open ourselves at the throat chakra which in turn gives our bodies permission to begin the healing process. When we ask for healing we put forth a conscious effort to become personally involved in our own positive growth and health, thus accepting personal responsibility for our healing and well-being. The request may also be made on any of the body levels such as the physical, mental/emotional, or spiritual.

2. There Must Be an Exchange of Energy for Services

Wellness has value, whether monetary or in-kind, and an exchange of some sort helps empower a person to take responsibility for their health. The healing energy belongs to the Universe. However, there needs to be a creative exchange from the recipient, to the practitioner whose time and services are being rendered balancing and healing. Energy exchange may be anything from money, to an exchange of services between the client and the practitioner.

Reiki practitioners offering healing services on a professional level do establish a fee. The fee sets a value on the service. Wellness, likewise, has a value, and ultimately reflects the feeling of worthiness and self-love of the person seeking to change their state of health.

The Twist™

Use common sense. The Reiki Precepts really boil down to making sure you are not taking advantage of anyone and that you are not forcing yourself or your views onto those who are susceptible. The precepts really stand on their own, but a possible third precept might be – Act with compassion. Every person on this world is deserving of compassionate understanding. If you act with compassion, you will most likely make sure your actions are ethical and sound.

The "Levels" of Reiki

The classification of Reiki into levels is a constant source of discussion and contention within the Reiki communities. Even within the same schools of Reiki and among Reiki masters, discussions on this topic can become quite heated. Opinions vary greatly as to which is the best way to divide up the learning process.

The Usui Method

First Degree

The Physical Level

How do you use your physical body – exercise, awareness, touch? What is the importance of water, outdoors, elements of earth to you?

The First Degree is the first level during which one receives the attunement to use the Reiki energy on the physical level. The attunement a student receives opens them to the Reiki energy and assists them in their healing sessions.

For a Reiki practitioner, nothing can be more important than being attuned to the Reiki energy. If they do not receive this attunement, they may still be able to practice using the techniques, but their energy will be scattered and unfocused in the Reiki methodology. They may still progress through the "Intuitive Energy Healing" modalities should they wish, but not through the Reiki tradition.

Besides the attunement, the student is taught the history, ethics, proper usage of, and hand positions for Reiki healing. In addition, they are provided an opportunity to practice all they have learned. They are taught both the science and metaphysics of Reiki, and given plenty of case histories to back up the theory.

They are also taught how to give self-treatments, to treat animals and plants, and to treat others in both crisis and chronic situations.

Interspersed with this are practical sessions wherein the students are given the opportunity to put things into practice and experience the Reiki firsthand with a partner.

The First Degree is often associated with just the physical healing of the body itself, however, it is understood that energy will go where it is needed.

Second Degree

The Mental/Emotional Level

> *How do you use your emotional energy?*
> *What fears are you working through – fear of*
> *death, fear of being left out, rejection, fear of*
> *loss, change, doubts, etc.? How can you open*
> *to more joy in your life and learn to express*
> *your emotions?*
>   *Are you able to use your mind to further*
> *your goals, or is your mind constantly in the*
> *way of you getting things done – too much*
> *worry, going over and over things, etc. Look at*
> *how you use your mind, and how you can use*
> *it for peace and spiritual evolution.*

In the Second Degree, the focus of this particular manual, the students are taught advanced techniques involving the use of symbols in their healing sessions as well as how to heal on the emotional and mental levels. The symbols are essentially energy patterns that, when utilized by someone initiated to them, enable practitioners to influence their lives in very powerful ways. The student is initiated to the symbols and then taught their many uses.

The symbols have other individual uses, such as energizing energy fields, harmonizing people and places, providing protection, and developing intuition. The level of Reiki energy in the hands is also increased through the attunement of Second Degree.

One of the most exciting Second Degree techniques is the treatment of people, or anything else at a distance. This is, of course, very different from the hands-on application of Reiki in First Degree, and has obvious practical benefits if you have loved ones or clients who live in other parts of the country or world.

The principles on how and why remote healing works are explained later on as are the many different methods. Once the principles are understood, the practical is easy.

Whereas First Degree Reiki is very straightforward in its physical application, the Second Degree is extremely eclectic and has expansive array of applications due to the mental and emotional level of healing. A person attuned to the Second Degree will be able to heal on both the physical and emotional or mental levels.

Third Degree

Also known as the Master Level
and the Spiritual Level

How important is your spiritual life? Are
you focused on it? Begin to look at your
soul's journey into the light, and at the path
of your spiritual evolution. How may you
evolve more spiritually? What is your
connection to the Divine? Do you believe in
a Divine force?

The Third Degree practitioner is considered to be a Master in the field of Reiki and is attuned to the spiritual nature of healing of energy.

The Third Degree student, once in touch with the higher levels of Reiki, can use them for any one of, or simultaneously for physical, emotional, or spiritual healing.

To qualify for Reiki Master training, one must demonstrate a strong ethical nature and have a sound background in the practical application of Reiki. One cannot become a Reiki Master simply because of interest or curiosity, or for intellectual reasons only.

Likewise, "blind faith" in the Reiki energy is also unacceptable as one must know how Reiki works from personal and hands-on experience in their own lives as well as from practical experience and observation of patients they have treated. Academic qualifications are not necessary, but can be helpful in the learning processes involved with lecture content.

The student must understand all the necessary theoretical knowledge taught by the Reiki teacher and be able to present it to others with full understanding, not just from memorization.

More important than the theoretical aspect is the development of the Spiritual side of the Reiki Master. The attunement process will open the student to the spiritual nature of the universe and energy and may even elevate the Reiki Master to be another level in their own personal development.

A Master is one who is able to find balance between all parts of the self, whether they be physical, emotional, or spiritual.

According to the Usui Method, this is also the teacher level. At this point a student should be able to teach the various levels of Reiki. In addition, the student is attuned to the teacher level.

The Twist™

Teacher Level

Many of the original schools of Reiki separated out the teacher level from the Master level as this was to be the level where students learned how to teach all they themselves have learned to their own students. By this point, students have received and been instructed in the methods of healing the physical body, the emotional or mental body, and the spiritual or ethereal body.

During the training students receive the knowledge and ability to perform each of the attunements for all the levels including the teacher level. Each attunement is then practiced and synthesized into the energy field of the student. This whole process varies between students according to their individual backgrounds. The average time taken is about one year.

Reiki Teachers are able to activate the Reiki energy in the hands of their students and can attune them to as high a level of awareness as they themselves have been attuned.

A teacher is merely a practitioner who is attuned to teach and who can attune others to any of the Reiki levels.

In ancient Japanese tradition this degree is not asked for, but may be offered by a teacher if the student is found worthy. If and when a teacher (Reiki Grandmaster) finds that the student (also known as a channel) has reached a satisfactory emotional, mental and spiritual level, she or he offers the teacher level (or by some traditions, Grand Mastership) to the student.

The number of days taken to learn this degree is not defined as most teachers require their students to train under them for a year or more in order to learn how to teacher others.

The Main Differences between The Various Levels

The Usui Method

Reiki I
1. Works on the physical level.
2. Colors from the chakras are utilized for healing.
3. Balance the Chakras
4. Self Reiki
5. Chair Reiki

Reiki II
1. Reiki II works on the mental and emotional level
2. Refinement of Balancing the Chakras
3. Use the 5 Kanji healing symbols that assist and enhance the healing.
4. Learn Distance healing.

Reiki III
1. Reiki III works on the spiritual, emotional, and physical levels.
2. Is a Master of Reiki
3. Learns to balance all three aspects of Energy.
4. Learns a couple additional symbols.

The Twist™

"The Twist™" method separates the Teacher from the Master level as follows:

Teacher
1. Can teach Reiki to others.
2. Can attune all three levels of Reiki

In the Twist™ tradition there are four levels or degrees in Reiki:
1.) The First Degree / Physical Level.
2.) The Second Degree / Emotional or Mental Level.
3.) The Third Degree / Spiritual Level (Master Level)
4.) The Teacher Degree

The rationale is simple: each of the degrees requires an attunement. The teacher level is no different. Often when one receives the Master attunement they are also receiving a "double dose" with the teacher attunement. Having both attunements at once can be overwhelming especially if a person is unaware they are receiving two attunements at once. Remember also there is a Twenty-One Day Cleanse for each and every level of Reiki which means that if you received both attunements at once you will undergo two cleanses at the same time.

With the teacher level broken out from the Master level a teacher can take their time to teach the Master the three Reiki levels, how to confer the attunements for each of the levels, and can attune the Master to the teacher level without worry of having to perform any other attunements.

The student is able to focus on the teachings for the Master level separate and apart from the teacher level, is able to fully grasp both levels without confusion, and receives each attunement separately thereby avoiding any compounding of issues which may arise, or without the "double dose" effect.

There is also an ethical component which comes into play with separating the two attunements. A Teacher should never force a student to undergo two attunements at once, AND a Teacher should assist the student in achieving a true mastery over the three levels of Reiki before the student moves on to the Teacher level.

Something else to consider is that not all Reiki Masters want to teach. If one wants to remain a practitioner, then the teaching part of Reiki is not needed and separating out the Teacher from the Master level honors the student's needs and intention.

It is likewise important to spend some time with the three levels of Reiki before moving on to the teaching level. This time frame is different for each person, but generally lasts for about a year.

Chapter 2: Hand Position Review

The Usui Method

The hand positions must follow the prescribed format and must not deviate from that prescribed form. The hand positions that follow are the prescribed form.

The Twist™

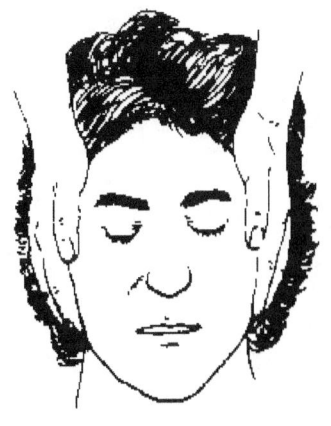

Several prominent Reiki Teachers have researched the original methods used by Dr. Usui and found he did not use hand positions the way we do today. The hand positions we use today were created by both Dr. Hayashi and later refined by Ms. Takata (Usui & Petter, 1999). Therefore, the hand positions below are only suggestions. You may use what feels most appropriate when working with clients. It is, however, very important to be respectful of the person while you are working on a client. Always explain to the client that any hand position can be changed or altered if it is uncomfortable. Seek feedback from your client regarding their comfort level and check for visual signals of discomfort.

Another thing to remember is if the client is uncomfortable with touch, you may work three to five inches above their body. The hand positions work regardless of physical touch or distance. The client's comfort and boundaries must be respected at all times regardless of the healer's knowledge, or intent. Remember, there is no place for ego so be sure to focus on your client's needs, not yours.

The Usui Method

The Byosen Scan

Scanning is a technique that involves feeling for the difference in a person's energy field. Hover your hands 3 to 5 inches above your client, with the fingers closed together and parallel to the client. Your hand should not be tensed, but relaxed as if gently resting on a balloon. Move your hands into one of the layers of the energy but still above the client. Pay close attention to any changes you feel in your hands as you pass your hands over the client from their head to their feet, like temperature changes, a feeling of pulling, drawing or pushing.

This is a technique that could require some practice so be patient the first few tries and repeat as often as necessary. If you still do not feel anything during the scan, proceed with the session knowing the energy will instinctively go where it's needed during the course of the session.

Once you have finished the scan, begin the hand positions.

The Front

Regardless of the method you are using, a practitioner should always begin a session with the client lying on their back, or what is known as the supine position.

While standing at the end of the table where the client's head is located, ask the client to take a couple of deep breaths and allow their body to relax more deeply each time they exhale. Remember to not push your hands down onto your client, but instead gently rest them in their respective positions. Check in with the client from time to time to see if the amount of pressure is comfortable.

1. Place your hands on the back of the client's head and hold the position for several minutes.
2. Place hands over or above the client's eyes (place a Kleenex over eyes first if requested).
3. Place hands over ears. (Slightly cup hands so you do not interfere with the client's hearing.)
4. Place hands in the throat position.
5. Place hands on shoulders.
6. Place hands forming a V (point of V away from you) on the heart center.
7. While standing at the side of the table by the client's arm:
   a) Place one hand on top of the upper arm &

slip one hand under the upper arm.

b) Cradle lower arm and hand. (For client's right arm - place your right arm with your hand under client's elbow and client's hand by your elbow and gently rest your left arm on top of client's with your left hand on top of the client's right hand.) If you have access to the other side of the table (in other words, if your table is not against a wall), then you can repeat the above process.

8. Place hands across the solar plexus.

9. Place one hand on each side of the hips. (This sends energy through the entire pelvic area but is not as invasive as the hands on top of the body below the waist.)

10. Place one hand in the center of each upper leg.

11. Place one hand on each knee.

12. Place one hand in the center of each lower leg.

13. While at the end of the table where the client's feet are located:

a) Place one hand on the top of each foot "OR"

b) place one hand on the top and one hand on the bottom of first one foot and then the other.

Sweeping the Front

Sweep the Client's Energy Field Three Times:

Start at the head area and working slowly towards the feet, sweep large circles moving in a clockwise direction above the client, to clear the energy of the person on whom you have just worked. When you are past the feet, have a clear mental intent that you are putting all that has been swept away into the White Light to be transmuted into positive energy which will not cause harm to others, then begin again at the head, working towards the feet for a total of three sweeps.

When you have finished sweeping your client's energy, gently and slowly, help your client turn over onto their stomach or what is known as the prone position.

The Back

While standing at the end of the table where the client's head is located:

1. Place hands gently on the back of the head. (Do not push down but gently rest your hands on the client. Check with the client to see if the amount of pressure is comfortable, until you get a feel for it.)
2. Place hands on back of the neck.
3. Place hands on the top of the right shoulder blade.
4. Place hands on the top of the left shoulder blade.
5. While standing at the side of the table by the client's arm:
6. Place hands on the top of the heart center.
7. Place hands on the top of the waist area.
8. Place one hand on each side of the hips. (This sends energy through the entire pelvic area but is not as invasive as the hands on top of the body below the waist.)
9. Place one hand in the center of each upper leg.
10. Place one hand on each knee.
11. Place one hand in the center of each lower leg.
12. While at the end of the table where the client's feet are located:
13. Place one hand on the top of each foot "OR" place one hand on the top and one hand on the bottom of first one foot and then the other.

The Twist™

In the Twist™ method, one is able to work directly on the affected area without having to go through the various hand positions. Additionally, connecting the various chakras and hand positions is not only permissible, but encouraged to help balance and smooth the energy throughout the body.

Sweeping the Back

Sweep the Client's Energy Field Three Times:

Just as you did for the front, start at the head area and working slowly towards the feet, sweep large circles moving in a clockwise direction above the client, to clear the energy of the person on whom you have just worked. When you are past the feet, have a clear mental intent that you are putting all that has been swept away into the White Light to be transmuted into positive energy which will not cause harm to others, then begin again at the head, working towards the feet for a total of three sweeps.

When you have finished sweeping your client's energy, normalize the chakras to help bring your client back to a grounded state and so you do not send them off open to all the energies of the universe.

Normalizing (Closing) the Chakras

Place both hands on top of the client's head. Leaving the left hand in place at the top of the head, move the right hand to normalize the 3rd eye, then the throat, the heart, solar plexus, spleen and root areas. Once you have done this with your right hand, leave your right hand on the root chakra. Now bring your left hand down through the chakras pushing the energy through the energy centers towards the root. Place your left hand on the root chakra and move your hands to the sides and off the body sending the excess energy into the ground.

Once you have completed all of these steps, bring your client's mind back to the space you are in and help them to a sitting position. Once they feel they have returned mentally and physically to the present, allow them to get off the table.

Both you and your client should drink some water to help move the toxins out of your systems, and help renew and refresh your balance. It will also help to ground both you and your client.

Wash Back

The Usui Method

Wash Back is a concept where the energy normally flows through the practitioner to, and through the client. The energy that comes from the client remains with the client and never affects the practitioner.

Wash Back allegedly occurs when the energy flows from the practitioner to the client, then for some reason reverses and flows back to the practitioner. In the traditional Usui method there is no such thing as "Wash Back", which means basically that neither the client nor the practitioner can pick up the other persons' issues.

The Twist™

Wash back is that empathic leftover feeling where the practitioner walks away from the session feeling the fullness of what the client is experiencing, whether positive or negative, as if they actually experienced the client's emotional or physical ailments. The most recent thought on "no wash back" is that if you are fully engaging in the Reiki energy, wash back is unavoidable, but easy to deal with and overcome.

There are many times during a session where a

Reiki practitioner must "check in" with the energy to see if more or less is needed in particular areas, or to determine when to move on to the next area. In fact, the very first thing a practitioner does in the course of a session is to scan the client and assess what is happening with the energy. This is the first moment where a practitioner opens themselves to connect with the energy of the client. During the session the practitioner should be checking to see if they are using too much or too little energy, or if they should be smoothing energy in certain areas or increasing it in other areas. Essentially there is an almost constant interaction between the energy of the practitioner and the energy of the client.

It is therefore essential that the practitioner has worked on, and continues to work on themselves by understanding who and what their emotional, physical, or other issues might be. The practitioner must be able to differentiate between their client's energy and their own without pause, and without question.

You should be fully present to your clients needs which means you MUST understand and come to terms with your own issues so you do not project them on your client. It is the responsibility of the healer to make sure they are also healed or in the process of healing before approaching the Reiki table or a client. If you are a model of health and well-being, then you will impart that sense of well-being to your client who will feel encouraged to continue seeking their own growth.

The moment a practitioner feels something out of the ordinary going on within them, they should deal with it then and there. If through the process of discernment the practitioner discovers the emotion or physical symptom is not theirs, then it needs to be released immediately. The practitioner should never allow the energy, which is not theirs, to take hold or it can become a permanent part of their person until formally released. With enough practice and self-knowledge the wash back effect will not be an issue, however, it is a concept which should not be ignored.

Releasing Energy Which Is Not Yours

There are two ways in which you can clear yourself of energy which may not be your own; one during the session, and one after the session. You do not need to do both methods, however, if after clearing yourself during a session you still find struggling with issues which are not your own, then you should also use the After a Session technique.

During a Session

During the course of a treatment, if you recognize something is happening which is different from what you felt when you started the treatment, it's time for you to sort out what is going on. For example if all of a sudden you feel angry, sad, or feel pain in your head, back or somewhere else in your body which you did not have before you began the session, check in with your client. Ask them if they have pain in their body or are feeling angry or sad. If they say yes, take a step back from the table to see if what you are sensing continues, or stops. If it continues, determine if what you are experiencing is yours or if you have taken on your client's energy. How is your body posture? Are you using proper body mechanics? When you feel confident to return to your client shake off the excess energy and continue the treatment. Shaking off the energy is simply a gentle shaking of your hands and arms, taking a deep breath in, then exhale with the intention of "letting go' of whatever energy you started absorbing. Finally, find your center, ground yourself, and then continue with the treatment or session.

If you still feel as if you have taken on your client's energy, excuse yourself and step away from the Reiki space for just a few moments, take a drink of water, and again breathe, find your center, ground yourself, and when you are ready return to working on the client. After the client has left take some time to understand what happened. Perhaps you have a similar issue as your client and something triggered within you which needs to be cleared. Make sure you take time for yourself and work through your own issues.

Remember you can also work above the client, not actually touching them which may be less intense for both you and the client.

After a Session

If you didn't notice the attachment to your client's energy during the session, or if you didn't deal with it at the time it occurred, then you can certainly clear yourself after the session is over. Determine what is, or isn't your energy, or issues. Take several clearing breaths, center yourself, shake your body, hands, arms, legs, and head. Drink some cold water, and then when you are ready release what isn't yours by recognizing yourself and your own energy from that of your client. Your intention should be that you release whatever is not your own "stuff", and that what is not yours go out from yourself to not harm anyone else. Check in with yourself by making sure you do not have any issues which you need to work through or release. Check to see if the physical or emotional sensation is still with you, and if not, take one more deep cleansing breath and release it with a sense of accomplishment. If you still feel yourself attached to the energy of your client, then perhaps you have keyed into something which may need healing within yourself. It may also be that simply might need to take a little longer to clear yourself. Sit with what is happening and what you are feeling and examine why you are feeling this way. Allow yourself to deal with, and work through whatever comes up. Then, when you have finished dealing with the issue, clear yourself again.

There is no right or wrong way to clear yourself of your client's energy. What is paramount is that you know what is, and what is not your own energy or your own issues so that when something comes up during the course of a Reiki session, you will know what is, and what is not your own energy

Chapter 3: Chakra Balancing Review

The word "Chakra" (pronounced shah'krah) comes from the Sanskrit meaning "Wheel" or "Circular Flow". A chakra will spin in relation to the energy level of the body energy system, either fast, slow, or somewhere in between.

A chakra is a wheel-like vortex, which according to traditional Indian medicine, is believed to exist at certain points or foci over a person's energy field.[5] They can be considered as mini tornadoes with the small ends hovering on, or just above the Chakra.

Chakras have also been described as "energy or force centers" or "whorls of energy" that emanate from a point on the physical body, and extend through all levels of the individual (physical, mental /emotional, and spiritual.) The chakras are considered to be the focal points for the reception and

---

5   Leadbeater, C. W. The Chakras. Wheaton: Theosophical House, 1927. Print.

transmission of all energy through a person or thing.[6]
There are believed to be seven main chakras that cover
the body, although there are many schools of thought
about the chakra system(s).

It is because of modern science that we know all
living things including humans, animals, and plants
give off some form of energy whether it is simple heat
energy, magnetic energy, frequency energy, or other
forms. These energies have direct influence on our
bodies, minds, and emotions, as well as other aspects
that we may not be aware.

The chakras exist in and around us all beginning at
the base of the spine or pelvic region (root chakra) and
moving up towards and out the top of the head (crown
chakra).

Chakras also coincide with the body's endocrine
system (Simpson, 1999; Judith, 2003; Stein, 1995; and
Nelan & Soldon, 2010). Each chakra has an influence
over the endocrine glands and internal organs in that
part of the body where the chakra is located and
sometimes covers a broader area.

The chakras are interrelated; one affects another.
The Root Chakra is the lowest of the 7 chakras and
spins the slowest or resonates at the lowest of the 7
vibration frequencies. The Crown Chakra is the highest

---

6   Cross, John R. Healing with the Chakra Energy System Acupressure,
    Bodywork, and Reflexology for Total Health. New York: North Atlantic
    Books, 2006. Print.

of the 7 chakras and spins the fastest and has the highest vibrational frequency (Nelan & Soldon, 2010)[7].

Each chakra has a different color. The colors are:
Red (Root)
Orange (Sacral)
Yellow (Solar Plexus)
Green (Heart)
Blue (Throat)
Indigo (Brow)
Violet (Crown)

Chakra Imbalances

Traditional Chinese medicine teaches the only cause of illness or disease is the congestion or blockage of energy.[8] When there is a blockage or imbalance in one part of the chakra system, it has a direct impact on all the other chakras.

In Reiki, imbalances in the chakras are known as energy blocks. When there is unreleased emotion such as fear, anger, or guilt accumulated from past experiences; or when there's been a lack of nurturing, love, and encouragement during the developmental

---

7   Soldon, J. C., & Nelan, K. J. (2010). *Reiki I: A manual* (2nd ed.). Glendale, WI: Sacred Wandering.

8   Carlson, Jodi L. *Complementary therapies and wellness practice essentials for holistic health care.* Upper Saddle River, N.J: Prentice Hall, 2003. Print.

period, the energy flows less freely to or from the chakras.

Whenever a person blocks an experience, they block the flow of energy to or from their chakras. The chakras become clogged with stagnated energy, spin irregularly or backwards, or can even become distorted or torn. When the chakras are functioning normally each one will remain open and spin properly to metabolize the particular energies needed from the universal energy field.

Imbalances can also occur when there is too much or too little energy flowing through the chakras. By understanding how each chakra affects a particular body function and life issue, it is possible to identify where a chakra is malfunctioning. Various techniques can then be used to balance the chakra system and restore homeostasis within individual - physically, emotionally, mentally, and spiritually.[9]

If there are imbalances within a certain chakra those imbalances can cause that chakra to close down and can also affect other chakras close to it to by either slowing them down or completely closing them. The chakra will remain closed until the issue surrounding the blockage is dealt with and cleared. Once cleared the energy flow is restored and a normal flow of energy cycles throughout the entire chakra system.

---

9   Rowden, Arline. "Chakras." Reiki II Class. Linette Corsten Reiki II
     Master, Milwaukee. Sept. 2001. Lecture.

Balancing the Chakras

There are many ways to balance the chakras and clear any energy blockages or imbalances. Some useful therapies and tools are: Healing the Inner Child, Intuitive/Spiritual Counseling, and Mental Health Counseling.

In addition there are also Love & Forgiveness Meditations, Releasing Meditations, Prayer, Sound Therapy, Massage, Yoga, Spiritual Healing, Reflexology, Reiki (the reason you are taking Reiki II), Meditation, Visualization, Healthy Diet & Exercise, Music, Aromatherapy, Flower Essences, Oils, Incense, Color, Affirmations, Introspection, and Journaling.

Chakras respond to sound, resonance frequencies, and color[10].

Chakra Name	Number	Note	Frequency (Hz)	Color
Crown	7	B	10k	Violet
Third Eye	6	A	05k	Indigo
Throat	5	G	880Hz	Blue
Heart	4	F	800Hz	Green
Solar Plexus	3	E	787Hz	Yellow
Sacral/Spleen	2	D	727Hz	Orange
Root	1	C	020 Hz	Red

10 Nelan, K. J., & Soldon, J. C. (2010). *Introduction to energywork, energy healing, and Reiki* (2nd ed.). Tucson, AZ: Sacred Wandering.

Chapter 4: Emotional Healing

"Watch your thoughts,
    they become words;
watch your words,
    they become actions;
watch your actions,
    they become habits;
watch your habits,
    they become character;
watch your character,
    for it becomes your destiny."

Frank Outlaw
(1977 May 18, San Antonio Light, What They're Saying,
Quote Page 7-B (NArch Page 28), Column 4, San
Antonio, Texas.)

Being a Reiki II practitioner is no better or worse
than being any of the other levels. This is not a more
powerful level than the previous, nor is it less
important than the next. You will still use the same
energy as before, but now be able to focus the healing
energy specific to mental and emotional healing.

What we think can become what we say and do.
Thinking, that is to say our mental/emotional process,
is itself a form of energy. Once we create something in
our minds or feel something within our beings (or
emotions) it becomes manifest in the world. This

energy is neither positive nor negative until we have actually done something with that thought or feeling. However, our thoughts, words, and actions can effect us on many levels. Things we have thought and said can be imprinted in our cells, muscles, and tissues within our bodies. Remember, all things are connected and all things originate from some form of energy.

The things we imprint upon may be conversations or disagreements we have had in the past, but the mental/emotional residue is left within us – imprinted deep within until we release that energy back into the universe.

Remembering back to our Reiki I training, energy imbalance can even happen when we are overly filled with positive energy. We must seek a balance to remain in a homeostatic state.

Reiki can help work through these issues to help determine what, if anything, needs to happen with these "old" issues. Do the old issues need to be held on to in order for us to learn new things or do they no longer serve us well and can be released? In either case, we are able to heal from past thoughts or feelings whether we knew those issues even existed.

Paramount in healing on the mental/emotional level is ensuring the client's needs, through their affirmation of their own intentions, is not only considered, but mandatory. The client's intentions are what should direct where the Reiki session will go.

Working from a mental/emotional level offers much in the way of helping sort through the thoughts and emotions that remain within a client to assist them with determining what they want to do about about those left over issues.

Caveat

Remember that ethics require us to only provide services for which we are qualified. Unless you are a qualified and licensed mental health professional, you should not be engaging in mental health counseling.

[11]

Working on the mental/emotional level is delicate work and key is remembering that we must take people where they are. Their particular realities might not be congruent with our own so we must seek to always understand the client's needs.

Thought and emotional energy are perhaps of the most powerful types due to the long lasting effects of both. One who has existed in a negative or positive frame experiences the world through that particular lens. What we, as practitioners, do or say can have long lasting repercussions – good or not so good.

---

11 Soldon, J. C., & Nelan, K. J. (2010). *Being an ethical Reiki practitioner* (2nd ed.). Glendale, WI: Sacred Wandering.

With a person who has existed in a positive frame, little needs to be done to help smooth or normalize their energy, however, a person who has existed in a negative way may need a bit more help.

Clients who have existed in that negative state can sometimes benefit from new perspectives, but here we must be careful to not project our own beliefs or needs onto the client. Sometimes simply restating what the client has said (re-framing) or carefully suggesting the client look for a more positive or nurturing solution can have a profound impact. Even more powerful is empowering the client to come up with their own solutions and finding ways to deal with their own issues. Occasionally we might have to refer out to qualified mental health professionals, but again, this is about the client and their highest good.

A Reiki II session will look identical to a Reiki I session with the only difference being that now the practitioner is more sensitive to the emotional or mental needs of the client. The hand positions, however, may take on new meanings.

One of the hand positions during a Reiki session is the practitioner placing their hands over a client's ears. The interpretation of the energy coming from the ears may be different on a mental/emotional level and can reveal a great deal about what is going on within a client. As a practitioner, you will need to interpret how the energy you are feeling may relate to what the client is feeling. An over abundance of energy coming from the ear or ears may indicate that something the client has heard or hears on a regular basis is affecting them in some way – good or not so good.

Working on a clients head can also offer an opportunity to sense if a client's mind is working overtime or if they are relaxed. If a client has a lot of activity going on in their head then that too is an opportunity to assist the client with sorting out what thoughts need to remain and what thoughts can be let go.

As with the physical level of healing, the practitioner should seek feed back from the client and ask about any thoughts, emotions, or conversations they have had that still remain within them. The client then makes the determination as to what, if anything they want to do about it. The Reiki practitioner should share with the client what they are sensing, but it is up to the client as to how they should proceed.

Working on or over a clients heart area is another place where the energy might take on a different meaning. High emotions can be felt in this area and as before the practitioner will need to interpret what they are feeling from the client. Again, the practitioner should tell the client what they are sensing/feeling and allow the the client to decide what needs to be done. Sometimes just an acknowledgement is all it takes to clear an emotion or feeling. Other times it can take some thought and lengthy processing on the part of the client to determine what to do with those feelings.

Sometimes the only way to work through physical issues is to first work through the mental/emotional ones. The mind greatly influences the body and studies have shown that often the body can heal if the mind allows for it. If a person believes they will never heal, then the consequence of that belief will equally manifest itself. Therefore, it is imperative that only the client's highest good be considered at each and every interval of treatment. A negative slip of the tongue may have drastic long term effects.

Perhaps one of the greatest tools in the Reiki II practitioner's tool bag is the use of Symbology. If the mind believes something is working, then the body is more prone to accepting what ever is being done. Sometimes physical healing is as simple as allowing the mind to relax to let the body do its thing. This is where using symbols in the healing process can have profound effect.

Chapter 5: The Reiki Symbols

What Are Symbols and Why Are They Used?

The dictionary defines symbol as (1) a sign or object accepted as recalling, typifying or representing a thing, quality or idea; or (2) a character, mark or sign standing for some process, idea, quality etc[12].

There are cultures which believe that sounds, thoughts, and intentions, can be drawn or thought of in such a way as to focus the mind, which of course then focuses the "power" or force of energy.

Reiki is no different in that regard, but there is great debate today as to the original symbols used, how many there were, or whether or not any documentation is available to support the multiplicity of claims regarding the now hundreds of symbols used in Reiki.

Every school or tradition seems to "discover" and use their own symbols within their individual practices, but in general practice, only 4 symbols were originally used by Ms. Takata when she brought Reiki to the West through her school in Hawaii. One of the symbols will not be discussed in this book as it pertains only to the master level.

As the other symbols became popular, they taught to

---

12 *Webster's new American dictionary.* "Symbol." Def. 1-3. New York: Smithmark, 1995. Print.

students before their attunements, and even used within the attunement.

So how does that relate to Reiki symbols? Remember there is only one source of energy, but that there are different qualities of that energy that can be called on and used for healing. Each Reiki symbol represents some qualities of an energy and is a tool or method of invoking various qualities of that energy.

Through the use of symbols in Reiki, you can send healing (energy) to any person (including yourself), place, situation or thing. You can also use the symbols to enhance hands on healing.

The Usui Method

Traditional Symbols:

The following three symbols are common to all traditions of Reiki for the Second Level.

The traditional Usui Method of using the symbols teaches that each symbol is repeated three times except for Hon Sha Ze Sho Nen, which is only drawn once, and are used for very specific reasons.

Mrs. Takata often made her students repeat writing the symbols on paper over and over again so they would achieve a high level of perfection drawing them in the air over their clients. Immediately after, she would destroy all copies of the symbols so they would never leave her school[13].

Please take care when using the following symbols, and only do so after you've been taught their full meaning and usage by a qualified Reiki Master/Teacher.

---

13 Hosak, Mark, and Walter Lübeck. *The Big Book of Reiki Symbols: The Spiritual Tradition of Symbols and Mantras of the Usui System of Natural Healing.* Twin Lakes, WI: Lotus, 2006. Print.

Hon Sha Ze Sho Nen:

- Pronounced: Hon (like won) Shaw Shay Show Nen
- Use: Distance Healing.
- When Used: At the very beginning of a distance healing session (do not use on a person directly).

Distant healing can bridge time and space, allowing you to send healing energy across a room, or around the world. This particular symbol is said to mean, "No Past, No Present, No future" suggesting that time and space are relative in healing.

You can use this symbol for long distance or to direct the energies to someone in the room. This is especially useful in treating children and animals, in treating yourself on areas you can not reach and when in public or anyplace where a hands on treatment might be impractical.

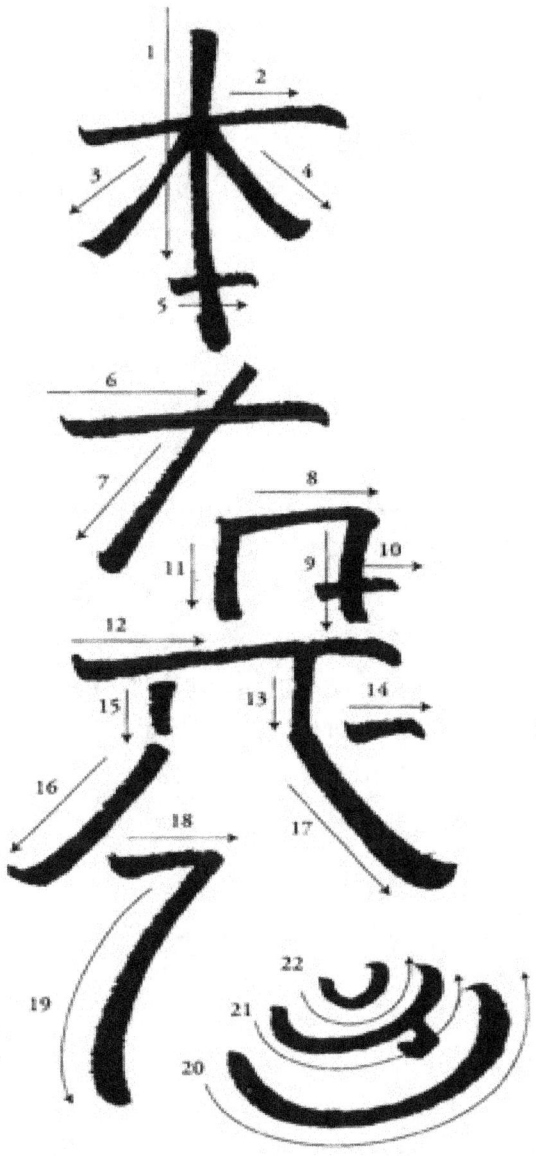

Hon-She-Ze-Sho-Nen
Distance healing, the Akashic Records, past–present–future

Sei He Ki:
- Pronounced: Say Hay Key
- Use: Mental and Emotional Healing.
- When Used: When ever needed during a session.

This mental/ emotional symbol is used to facilitate emotional and mental healing during a Reiki session and is defined as: "As above, so below", or "Divinity and People coming together". This is a very mild symbol and is not as strong as others. It nurtures and helps a person come to terms with the emotional, or mental blockage.

It is said to work on the subconscious. Some teachers use it on the chakras four, five, six and seven only, though some practitioners use it on all positions. The mental or emotional healing symbol helps to balance the right and left sides of the brain, and is often used for healing unwanted habits and for an emotional release. It clears a person, room and helps in mental issues as well.

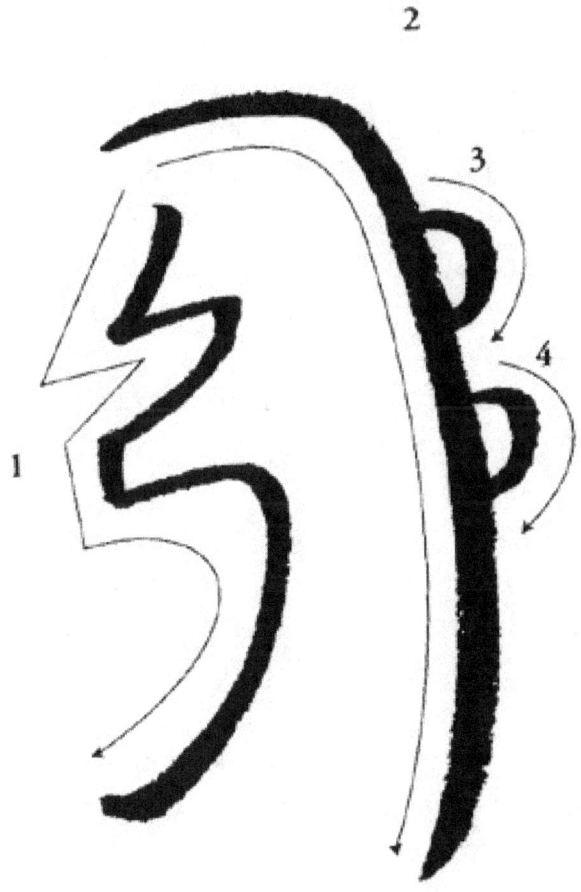

Sei-He-Ki
Emotional healing, purification, protection, and clearing

Cho Ku Rei:
- Pronounced: Show Coo (Like moo) Ray
- Use: To Increase or Decrease Energy Flow
- When Used: When ever needed during a session.

Cho Ku Rei is the symbol to either increase the flow of Reiki or decrease the flow of energy depending on how you draw the symbol. It concentrates the energy in a focused area by calling all the energy into the specific location.

This energy calls in higher universal energy and accelerates Reiki from low to high and gives greater power and focus to the energy.

Power boost is used with the other energies as well as by itself during all treatments hands on or distance.

Cho Ku Rei can also be used to empower other symbols or to lessen their effects depending on the needs of the client.

The symbol can be drawn clockwise to increase the flow of energy during a session or to enhance or empower another symbol. If the symbol is drawn counter-clockwise, it can be used to unblock stagnant energy or decrease the flow of energy.

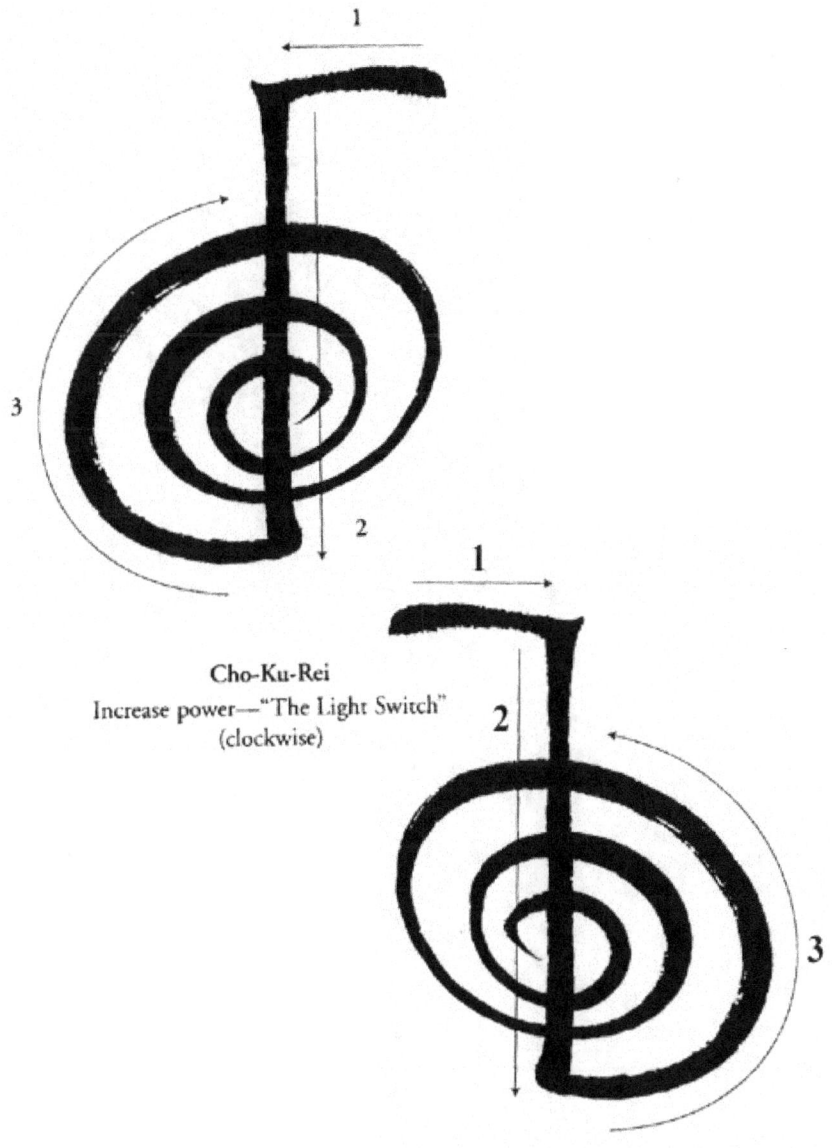

Cho-Ku-Rei
Increase power—"The Light Switch"
(clockwise)

Cho-Ku-Rei
To decrease energy - often used to help bring
down fever and inflammation.
Counter-clockwise

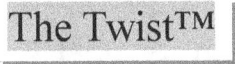

The Twist™

Non-Traditional Symbols

There are many symbols existing from a wide range of traditions other than the Usui based Reiki methods. Entire books have been dedicated to the study of Reiki symbols' and it is greatly suggested that each student make a concerted effort to discover for themselves if they feel drawn to particular symbols. Reiki is not an exact science and the practitioner should feel free to experiment and see what works best for the client. It is also important to keep up with new and major discoveries in Reiki. The Big Book of Symbols II[14] suggests that a practitioner should study the symbols from all traditions so as to gain a comprehensive understanding of the Reiki community as a whole. Regardless of the tradition, it is important to engage in continuing education in the field. Reiki symbology is only one of many areas of study available to the practitioner.

In the "The Twist™" tradition, if the practitioner feels the symbols only need to be drawn once, then draw them only once. If the practitioner feels they need to be drawn multiple times, then do so.

---

14 Hosak, Mark, and Walter Lübeck. *The Big Book of Reiki Symbols: The Spiritual Tradition of Symbols and Mantras of the Usui System of Natural Healing.* Twin Lakes, WI: Lotus, 2006. Print.

The following symbols, while not part of the original tradition, are included here for the benefit of both the client and the student. The following symbols have been shown to work well within the traditional Usui methodology.

Zonar:
- Pronounced: Zoe Nar
- Use: To Increase Mental or Emotional Clarity.
- When Used: Only when a deep healing needs to take place.

Zonar is a very powerful symbol which should be used sparingly. It means "Infinity", or "Eternity" and helps us create clarity and open our hearts to compassion. Our awareness broadens while Zonar opens dimensions of our understanding. It connects us to loving compassionate energy. It also heals past issues.

It connects us to loving and compassionate energy. It also heals past issues: such as child abuse, addictions fears, or phobias. It helps release some suppressed traumatic issues, and helps the body clear memories of the past that may still exist within the subconscious.

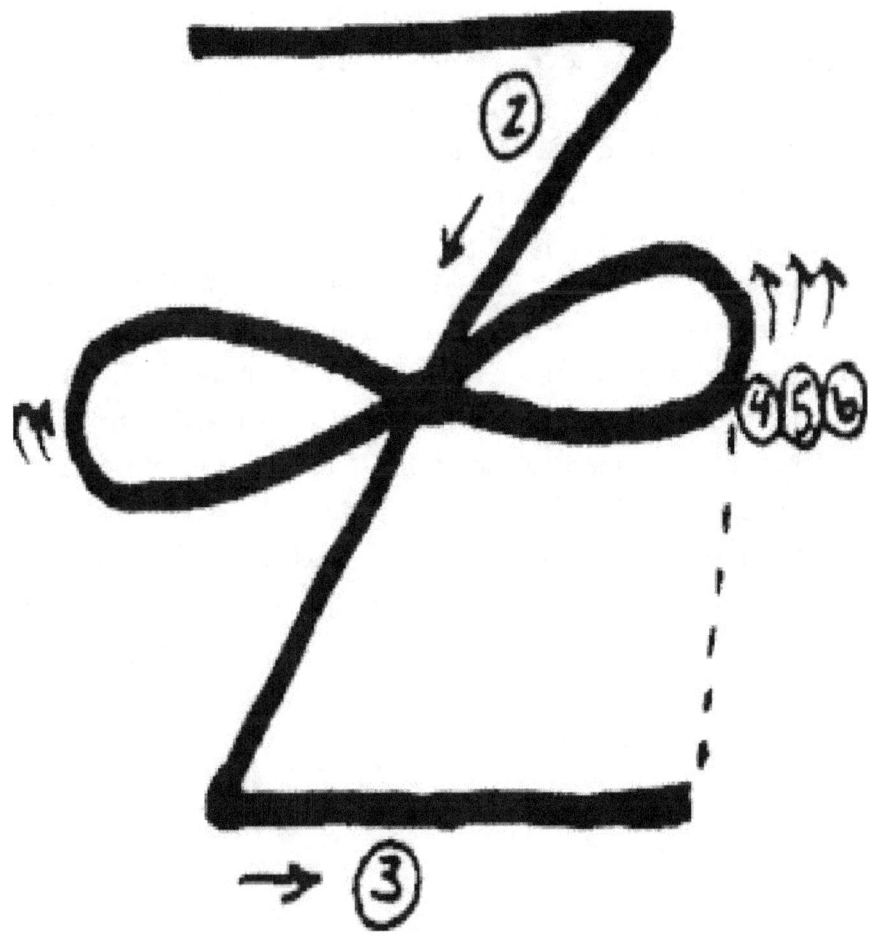

Harth:
- Pronounced: Hearth (just like the fireplace.)
- Use: To heal issues of the heart and emotions.
- When Used: During emotional or heart healing.

Harth means love, truth, beauty, harmony and balance and represents infinite compassion. Harth restores our love of life as it is used to heal issues of the heart, replacing fear, anger and sadness with love.

Harth can bring healing in the area of relationships, unmet hopes, dreams or even expectations in love. Some "love" relationships we enter into bring about a learning process from each other. If we have each learned all we needed from the relationship it may end. Harth can bring the healing we need to move on. It brings compassion for ourselves and others.

Harth can also facilitate an internal change you may wish to make. Look seriously at what you wish changed, then use the symbol while thinking of the replacement for what you wish changed.

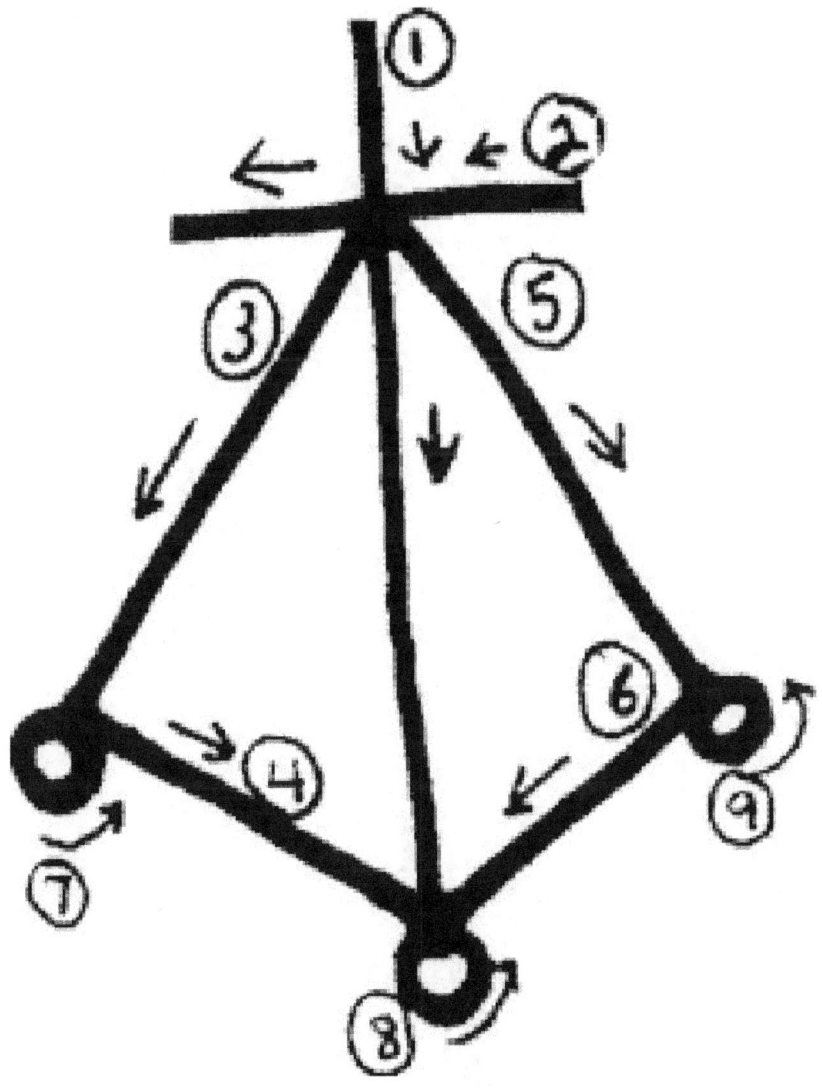

Chapter 6: Distance Healing

What is Distance Healing?

Since energy knows no boundaries or limitations, it can go wherever it is needed, therefore, anyone can be treated from a distance. This may be a new concept for some of you, but just think about it and it truly does make sense.

The Reiki energy will move over great distances so you can effectively give someone a Reiki healing when you are in the next room, or even across State lines. If you chose to, you could heal someone on the other side of the world.

Why should we want to use distance healing? Well, first of all, people who cannot be physically with you, like a family member or friend living far away, may request a healing and you don't have to be in the same room to accommodate their needs.

Second for people who cannot sit or lie still for a treatment, like children and animals, you can sit in the same room with them and give them treatments using remote techniques.

Third for a person's body-parts which hurt too much to be touched, like burns, you can work above them, or work on a substitute which represents the client.

Distance healing is also usually done in a relatively short amount of time. Since the healing is done remotely, it takes less time than if the client were present.

And finally, it is a convenient way to treat yourself (putting your hands on your back for instance is not really comfortable).

In distance healing we make use of something to represent the person or thing needing the healing or Reiki energy such as a photograph, teddy bear, doll, or anything really so long as it can be imbued with the identity of the person or thing it is meant to represent.

Another well known method is projecting the image someone or something on your upper leg using just your imagination; in this example the knee represents the head of the person, the upper thigh their legs and feet of the person, and so on. It may sound strange and unbelievable, but thousands of people work this way with great results.

It encompasses a visualization process of who the recipient is receiving the treatment.

With distance healing, we have greater need of using the symbols; the number of symbols is up to the practitioner, but at the very least you will need to use the distance symbol (Hon Sha Ze Sho Nen) which travels through time and space, the power symbol (Cho Ku Rei), and Sei He Ki for mental and, or emotional healing.

Another reason for using the Reiki symbols with your visualizations, or to the healing thoughts you send out is that the Reiki symbols will make your work that much more effective.

Of course you can write down affirmations or your wishes on a piece of paper accompanied by the Reiki symbols and hold it between your hands, or you can use your hands to send Reiki to a person either present or far away just by visualizing the symbols in your mind and placing the palms of your hands outwards.

In each of these cases, your own intention must match that of the person receiving the energy. We must always seek permission for sending the energy, and if someone has requested remote healing, it is generally a good idea to try and set up a mutual time where you both can be in stillness, and quiet to send and receive the energy.

Whenever we send healing to someone else, whether it's hands on or distance, the person needs to ask (remember it's one of the precepts). It is vital that you know whether or not the person you are sending healing to has asked for the healing or is open to receiving remote healing. If they don't want it for whatever reason and you send them healing anyway, be aware that you might be forcing your own will and / or energy on someone else.

The Method

1. Distance healing always begins by using the hon sha ze sho nen symbol which helps open the doorway for remote healing. The symbol can be drawn either in the air or over the substitute and is only drawn once.
2. State the intention of the individual needing the healing. This is where it is generally a good idea to try to sit down to do the healing at the same time as the person needing the healing.
3. Begin the same hand positions over the substitute that you would use on the client as if they were physically present. - The substitute is either your leg, a teddy bear, another person, or other appropriate representation of the person needing the healing.
4. - If there is a particular need or if the healing is for a specific reason, then you can focus solely on that area without having to do a complete session.
5. Close as you would as if your client was present by sweeping the energy and then normalizing the chakras.
6. Center and ground yourself after your session and don't for get to drink lots of water.

Chapter 7: Final Words

The Attunement

This is the process by which the Reiki Teacher (often called Reiki Master) passes on the ability to channel Reiki energy. This involves a process of clearing any blocks to Reiki (chi) in your physical and ethereal body connecting you to the ability to run Reiki energy through your hands. This process opens the crown, third-eye or brow, throat, heart, and palm chakras and creates a special link between the student and the Reiki source.

The Reiki attunement is a powerful spiritual experience. The attunement energies are channeled into the student through the Reiki Teacher/Master.

The attunement can also increase intuitive/psychic sensitivity. Students often report experiences involving: opening of the third eye, increased intuitive awareness, and other intuitive/psychic abilities after receiving a Reiki attunement.

Once you have received a Reiki attunement, you will have Reiki for the remainder of your life. It does not wear off and you can never lose it. While one attunement is all you need for each level, additional attunements bring benefit.

The student is asked to sit down in a chair, with their feet flat on the floor with their hands placed palms together. Their eyes may be open or closed. The Reiki Teacher stands in front of the student and then stands behind the student completing a ritual that involves the empowering of the student to direct the healing energy.

The student should wear loose comfortable clothing and shoes that easily be removed if asked to do so.

During the attunement some people may or may not experience feelings of the energy moving through or around them. Others may see colors or forms, symbols, hear sounds, or have physical sensations. Still others do not have any unusual sensations at all this does not make a difference in their ability to use Reiki.

Many people can feel the attunement as it is done, as heat or waves of energy flowing into their body or they may see light etc. Some people do not have any such experience at all other than perhaps feeling both more relaxed and energized than usual. Most people, but not all, who regularly feel subtle energies are able to feel some of the energy coming in.

After the Attunement

The Reiki attunement can start a cleansing process that affects the physical body as well as the mind and emotions. Toxins that have been stored in the body may be released along with feelings and thought patterns that are no longer useful.   It is recommended that you drink lots of water after an attunement. Attunements and treatments may (rarely) cause physical detoxification.

Anyone one receiving Reiki treatments and or attunements is encouraged to drink lots of water and reminded that in some rare cases the release of toxins and/or energetic or physical realignments will cause them to feel worse for a short time before they feel better.

Please contact your Reiki Teacher if you have some unusual experience which you feel may related to your attunement. Any severe or continuing unusual discomfort should be referred to an appropriate medical professional because it could possibly not be related to the attunement at all.

After the attunement you will want to practice activating and using your Reiki as soon as you can. You may get the sensations of feeling heat in your hands or sensing energy flow or not. Sometimes it takes a bit of practice to get the used to running the Reiki energy.

The 21 Day Cleansing Process

After the attunement process in each of the three degrees, the student will undergo a Twenty-One day cleansing process. This is a time when the body detoxifies, balances, and integrates the energies from the attunement. The cleansing is different for each person, but for everyone, the cycle starts on the day of the attunement with the root chakra, on day two, the spleen or sacral chakra, on day three the solar plexus, day four the heart, day five the throat, day six the brow or third eye, and day seven the crown.

In week two the cycle starts over with the root on day eight and continues each day until the crown on day fourteen then the cycle again continues for week three on day fifteen through twenty-one. Week one focuses on physical healing, week two on emotional or mental healing, and week three on spiritual healing. This cleansing process came from the tradition of Dr. Usui's fast on Mt. Kurama and being on mountain for twenty-one days cleansing his own seven chakras.

For some, physical symptoms may surface; a pain, cough, headache, or even flu-like symptoms. For others nothing noticeable will surface during the Twenty-One day cleanse. It can be helpful to keep a journal of what you are feeling each day. Breathing exercises and drinking lots of water to flush toxins can be helpful as well as eating lighter meals which include vegetables, fruits, and juices.

For some, emotions may surface, such as sadness, grief, anger, intense happiness, joy, or even euphoria as well as other emotions. This is not at all unusual. Emotional releases can clear issues that have been held in for some time and may also release old blockages. This is a very positive occurrence; just be patient and you will work through it.

Old thought patterns may surface and you may notice your old way of thinking doesn't serve you any longer. Be aware of those thoughts; evaluate whether or not they continue to represent who you are and how you think. Do you still think in those ways, or have new thoughts replaced old bad habits? Keep what feels right and pure, and release the rest never to harm you again.

Be gentle with yourself, not judging or condemning, but recognizing that was "where you were" and now you are somewhere else. Let go of those old thoughts and create new thoughts, using affirmations daily to achieve what you are becoming or what you wish to become.

On the spiritual level, you may question old beliefs. The key here is to find what now fits your "belief" system. Reconcile your beliefs and find peace with what now fits who you are and your own individual growth.

We continue to grow, modify, and change who and what we are. We are not stagnant beings, but dynamic and intelligent. Don't dismiss what is going on inside you, but embrace the changes and move through them becoming stronger and more aware of how you relate to the energy around you.

How long must I wait for the next attunement?

The answer will be different for each person. For some it may be years, for others months and still others will want it right away. There should be a minimum of 21 days before an additional attunement should be received.

To receive the Reiki III, or the Master attunement, we recommend waiting at least six months after a Reiki II initiation, so that there is time to fully incorporate the healing energy, the 21 Day Cleanse, and to allow time to practice on yourself and others. There are very deep responsibilities that accompany the Reiki Master throughout their life and time must be taken to fully appreciate the subtleties Reiki has to offer. This is where time is needed to just "Be Reiki".

Today we know everything is composed of energy, and so everything has a vibration. As your own vibration rises, so too will your awareness of your greater connection to the Universal flow of Energy.

May you continue to, Be Reiki.

The Authors

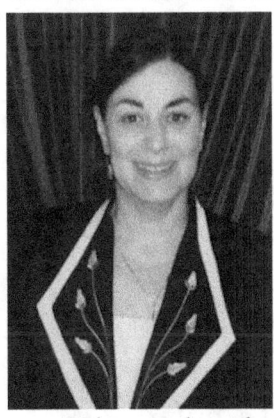

Janet C. Soldon, MA, RM/T, Retired LSW

Janet Soldon is a Master / Teacher of the Usui Shiki Rhoyo method of Reiki, as well as an intuitive energy practitioner, and has been an active practitioner for the past 26 years.

Prior to her healing practice Jan worked as a Social Worker/Supervisor in Child Welfare and Protective services in Milwaukee, which was a strong foundation for not only for her healing work, but also helping her engage in self-care and find balance.

In 2004, Jan and her husband Ken moved to Tucson, Arizona where she worked as a Reiki Master / Teacher and practitioner for seven and a half years. In addition to private practice, Jan and her husband were instrumental in developing and implementing the wellness education component of the Therapeutic Massage Program at Pima Community College. She developed and taught the following wellness education classes there for six years:

- Introduction to Reiki/Energy
- Reiki I and II
- Introduction to Complementary and Alternative Medicine

- Self-Care (including Healing the Inner Child)
- Stress Management

She collaborated with her husband to write and publish five books/manuals:
- Introduction to Reiki/Energywork
- Reiki I
- Reiki II
- Reiki III
- Being an Ethical Reiki practitioner

She returned to Milwaukee in 2011 and is currently working within a Chiropractic Wellness Center. As a part of her personal practice and philosophy, she helps empower and guide others to their own healing. She believes in client centered care with collaboration between client and practitioner, as well as providing a safe environment for her clients. She places a heavy emphasis on confidentiality, professionalism, and ethics.

Jan began her research into alternative and complementary medicines during her own cancer experience. It was then that she discovered various types of healing practices including Reiki, Intuitive Energy Work, Massage, Craniosacral, Reflexology, Aromatherapy, Acupuncture, Meditation and Chiropractic.

Jan is an experienced meditation guide and has conducted meditation sessions for beginning and intermediate levels.

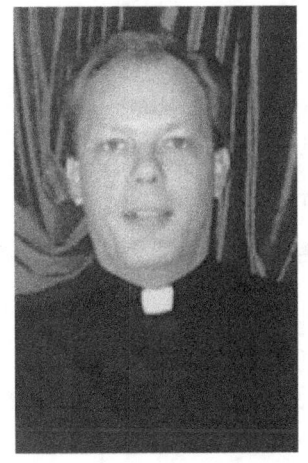

Rev. Kenneth J. Nelan, OPoc

Fr. Ken is a Master / Teacher of Reiki now living in the greater Milwaukee area. His path in the field of Energy Healing began in the mid 1980's and he now has over 30 years of experience.

Introduction to Energy, Reiki I and Reiki II are just a few of the classes Ken taught with his wife Jan at Pima Community College in Arizona. He also taught the Business Management for Body Workers and other Massage Professionals and was one of the voices of professionalism and ethics in the Therapeutic Massage program.

Together with his wife, Fr. Ken wrote:

- Introduction to Reiki/Energywork
- Reiki I
- Reiki II
- Reiki III
- Being an Ethical Reiki practitioner

They are also collaborating on a comprehensive teaching manual.

Fr. Ken is also an experienced meditation guide and retreat master for both religious and secular needs.

Fr. Ken was ordained a catholic priest in the Independent Catholic Movement in 2001 and was recently named to the Servant General for the Order of Preachers, Old Catholic and Vicar General for the Diocese of St. Catherine of Siena under the International Old Catholic Churches.

He works with his wife in a very successful private practice and has turned to writing in his spare time to help others come to a more complete view of the self, energy, and healing.

Recently, Fr. Ken returned to school to complete his education. He graduated with a BA in Latin American, Caribbean, and U.S. Latino Studies with a minor in Community Engagement and Education from the University of Wisconsin – Milwaukee. Early 2014 he was accepted into the Master's of Educational Psychology program where he studies Community Counseling. It is his hope to obtain his Licensed Professional Counselor license in both Wisconsin and South Carolina.

Other Publications

Janet Soldon and Kenneth Nelan have written manuals for Social Work and other industries, but have turned their collective focus to Energy Work.

The following books are currently available:

Introduction to Energy Healing and Reiki

Reiki I: A Manual

Reiki II: A Manual

Reiki III: A Manual

Being an Ethical Reiki Practitioner

The following books are currently in production:

Reiki for Massage Chair

Teaching Reiki

For more information about Janet Soldon or Kenneth Nelan, visit their website at:
http://www.sacredwandering.com

Recommended Reading

The following is a list of books we highly recommend.

Friesen, Corinne. *Reiki Symbols Cards (Reiki Learning Series)*. Print.
ISBN: 9781897266229

Fulton, Elizabeth, and Kathleen Prasad. *Animal Reiki Using Energy to Heal the Animals in Your Life*. New York: Ulysses, 2006. Print.
ISBN: 9781569755280

Horan, Paula. *Empowerment Through Reiki (Shangri-La Series)*. New York: Lotus, 1990. Print.
ISBN: 9780941524841

Hosak, Mark And Luebeck,Walter. *Big Book of Reiki Symbols, The*. New York: Lotus, 2006. Print.
ISBN: 9780914955641

Judith, A. (2003). Chakra Balancing Workbook. Bolder, CO: Sounds True.
ISBN: 1591790883

Nelan, K. J., & Soldon, J. C. (2010). *Introduction to energywork, energy healing, and Reiki* (2nd ed.). Tucson, AZ: Sacred Wandering.
ISBN: 9781456342562

Rand, William Lee. *The Reiki Touch complete home learning system*. Riverside: Sounds True, 2005. Print. ISBN: 9781591793700

Simpson, L. (1999). The book of chakra healing. New York: Sterling. ISBN: 0806920971

Soldon, J. C., & Nelan, K. J. (2010). *Being an ethical Reiki practitioner* (2nd ed.). Glendale, WI: Sacred Wandering. ISBN: 9781460926086

Soldon, J. C., & Nelan, K. J. (2010). *Reiki I: A manual* (2nd ed.). Glendale, WI: Sacred Wandering. ISBN: 9781456310707

Soldon, J. C., & Nelan, K. J. (2010). *Reiki III: A manual* (2nd ed.). Glendale, WI: Sacred Wandering. ISBN: 9781475189636

Stein, Diane. *Essential Reiki a complete guide to an ancient healing art*. Freedom, CA: Crossing, 1995. Print. ISBN: 0895947366

Usui, Mikao, and Frank Arjava Petter. *The Original Reiki Handbook*. New York: Lotus, 1999. Print. ISBN: 9780914955573

My Own Notes:

www.ingramcontent.com/pod-product-compliance
Lightning Source LLC
Chambersburg PA
CBHW070537290526
45790CB00002B/533